This Fitness Journal BELONGS TO:

●●●●●●●●●●●●●●●●

DEDICATION

This book is dedicated to all the amazing people who love fitness
out there!

You are my inspiration in producing books and I'm excited
to help in the planning of incorporating fitness into your day around the world!

How to Use this ULTIMATE Fitness Planner Notebook:

The purpose of this Fitness Workout Planner is to keep all your various fitness workout activities and ideas organized in one easy to find spot.

Here are some simple guidelines to follow so you can make the most of using this book:

1. The first "My Fitness Journal" section is for you to write the before and after measurements of your body so that you can track your fitness adventures.

2. Most ideas are inspired by something we have seen. Use the "12 Month Tracker" section to write down your measurements and weight loss so you can go back there to be reminded later.

3. The "Workout Ideas" section is for you to write out which workout ideas and exercises you preferred and a space for notes are included.

4. Some ideas require listing them out, the "Workout Tracker" section is great for describing where your favorite activity, time, sets, reps, and calories burned.

5. Flip the page over and this is where your Fitness Tracker information begins.

6. The "January Snapshot" section is so you can list out your goals, what I want to work on, how I will reach my goals and be inspired to add to your fitness journal and for each month after that.

7. And finally pages with a "Food Journal" section for you to make entries about each meal and track glasses of water taken in by checking them off, and a special place for any notes for making wishes come true...and much much more.

Have fun!

My Fitness JOURNEY

DATE

Keep track of your measurements every week and include photos.

BEFORE	AFTER

● ● ● ● ● ● ● ● ● ● ● ● ●

ARMS:

CHEST:

WAIST:

HIPS:

THIGHS:

BICEP:

WEIGHT:

12-Month TRACKER

Use this 12-month tracker to document your measurements and weight loss progress. Record your weight in the box below.

MONTH 1

WEIGHT:

	MEASUREMENT	NOTES
ARMS		
CHEST		
WAIST		
HIPS		
THIGHS		
BICEP		
SHOULDERS		

MONTH 2

WEIGHT:

	MEASUREMENT	NOTES
ARMS		
CHEST		
WAIST		
HIPS		
THIGHS		
BICEP		
SHOULDERS		

NOTES

12-Month TRACKER

Use this 12-month tracker to document your measurements and weight loss progress. Record your weight in the box below.

MONTH 3

WEIGHT:

	MEASUREMENT	NOTES
ARMS		
CHEST		
WAIST		
HIPS		
THIGHS		
BICEP		
SHOULDERS		

MONTH 4

WEIGHT:

	MEASUREMENT	NOTES
ARMS		
CHEST		
WAIST		
HIPS		
THIGHS		
BICEP		
SHOULDERS		

NOTES

12-Month TRACKER

Use this 12-month tracker to document your measurements and weight loss progress. Record your weight in the box below.

MONTH 5 — WEIGHT:

	MEASUREMENT	NOTES
ARMS		
CHEST		
WAIST		
HIPS		
THIGHS		
BICEP		
SHOULDERS		

MONTH 6 — WEIGHT:

	MEASUREMENT	NOTES
ARMS		
CHEST		
WAIST		
HIPS		
THIGHS		
BICEP		
SHOULDERS		

NOTES

12-Month TRACKER

Use this 12-month tracker to document your measurements and weight loss progress. Record your weight in the box below.

MONTH 7

WEIGHT:

	MEASUREMENT	NOTES
ARMS		
CHEST		
WAIST		
HIPS		
THIGHS		
BICEP		
SHOULDERS		

MONTH 8

WEIGHT:

	MEASUREMENT	NOTES
ARMS		
CHEST		
WAIST		
HIPS		
THIGHS		
BICEP		
SHOULDERS		

NOTES

12-Month TRACKER

Use this 12-month tracker to document your measurements and weight loss progress. Record your weight in the box below.

MONTH 9

WEIGHT:

	MEASUREMENT	NOTES
ARMS		
CHEST		
WAIST		
HIPS		
THIGHS		
BICEP		
SHOULDERS		

MONTH 10

WEIGHT:

	MEASUREMENT	NOTES
ARMS		
CHEST		
WAIST		
HIPS		
THIGHS		
BICEP		
SHOULDERS		

NOTES

12-Month TRACKER

Use this 12-month tracker to document your measurements and weight loss progress. Record your weight in the box below.

MONTH 11

WEIGHT:

	MEASUREMENT	NOTES
ARMS		
CHEST		
WAIST		
HIPS		
THIGHS		
BICEP		
SHOULDERS		

MONTH 12

WEIGHT:

	MEASUREMENT	NOTES
ARMS		
CHEST		
WAIST		
HIPS		
THIGHS		
BICEP		
SHOULDERS		

NOTES

Workout IDEAS

EXERCISE / WORK OUT IDEAS **NOTES**

Workout TRACKER

DATE

ACTIVITY	TIME	SETS	REPS	WT.	CAL BURNED

DATE

Workout TRACKER

ACTIVITY	TIME	SETS	REPS	WT.	CAL BURNED

DATE

Workout TRACKER

ACTIVITY	TIME	SETS	REPS	WT.	CAL BURNED

January SNAPSHOT

JANUARY FITNESS GOALS

WHAT I WANT TO WORK ON

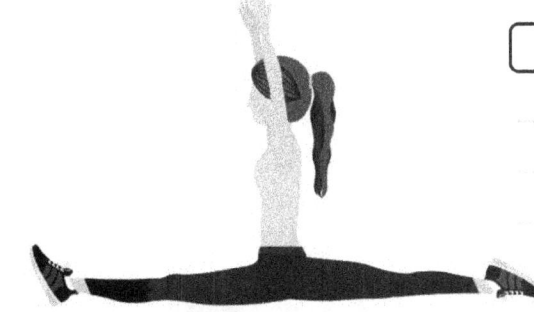

HOW I WILL REACH MY GOAL

THERE ARE NO Shortcuts TO ANY - PLACE - WORTH GOING

TOP FOCUS OF THE MONTH

NOTES

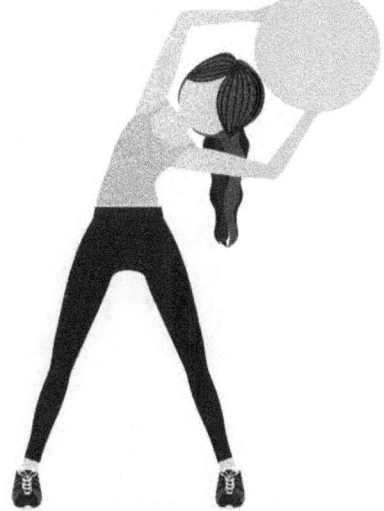

My Food JOURNAL

BREAKFAST:

LUNCH:

DINNER:

CALORIE GOAL **DATE**

My Food DIARY

MEAL	DESCRIPTION	CALORIES	CARBS

Monthly Fitness LOG

FITNESS DIARY

TOP FITNESS GOALS

ACHIEVE

NOTES

Don't forget to hydrate!

MEAL PLAN

BREAKFAST	LUNCH	DINNER

Weekly OVERVIEW

● ● ● ● ● ● ● ● ● ● ● ● ● ● ●

MONDAY

TUESDAY

WEDNESDAY

THURSDAY

FRIDAY

SATURDAY

SUNDAY

NOTES

Food & Exercise LOG

	BREAKFAST	LUNCH	DINNER	SNACKS	EXERCISE
M					
T					
W					
T					
F					
S					
S					

Food & Exercise LOG

	BREAKFAST	LUNCH	DINNER	SNACKS	EXERCISE
M					
T					
W					
T					
F					
S					
S					

Food & Exercise LOG

M | BREAKFAST | LUNCH | DINNER | SNACKS | EXERCISE

T | BREAKFAST | LUNCH | DINNER | SNACKS | EXERCISE

W | BREAKFAST | LUNCH | DINNER | SNACKS | EXERCISE

T | BREAKFAST | LUNCH | DINNER | SNACKS | EXERCISE

F | BREAKFAST | LUNCH | DINNER | SNACKS | EXERCISE

S | BREAKFAST | LUNCH | DINNER | SNACKS | EXERCISE

S | BREAKFAST | LUNCH | DINNER | SNACKS | EXERCISE

Food & Exercise LOG

M | BREAKFAST | LUNCH | DINNER | SNACKS | EXERCISE

T | BREAKFAST | LUNCH | DINNER | SNACKS | EXERCISE

W | BREAKFAST | LUNCH | DINNER | SNACKS | EXERCISE

T | BREAKFAST | LUNCH | DINNER | SNACKS | EXERCISE

F | BREAKFAST | LUNCH | DINNER | SNACKS | EXERCISE

S | BREAKFAST | LUNCH | DINNER | SNACKS | EXERCISE

S | BREAKFAST | LUNCH | DINNER | SNACKS | EXERCISE

January SNAPSHOT

FITNESS PROGRESS PHOTO

MY TOP ACCOMPLISHMENT THIS MONTH

_____
_____
_____
_____
_____

WHAT I HAVE LEARNED

_____
_____
_____

PAIN IS ONLY TEMPORARY BUT VICTORY IS FOREVER

SET YOUR GOALS HIGH AND DON'T STOP TILL YOU GET THERE

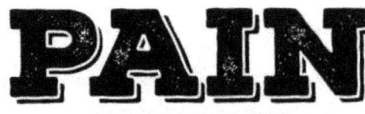

WHAT TO DO NEXT MONTH

_____
_____
_____

February SNAPSHOT

FEBRUARY FITNESS GOALS

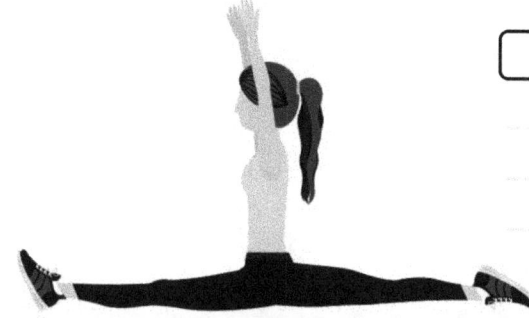

WHAT I WANT TO WORK ON

HOW I WILL REACH MY GOAL

THERE ARE NO Shortcuts TO ANY - PLACE - WORTH GOING

TOP FOCUS OF THE MONTH

NOTES

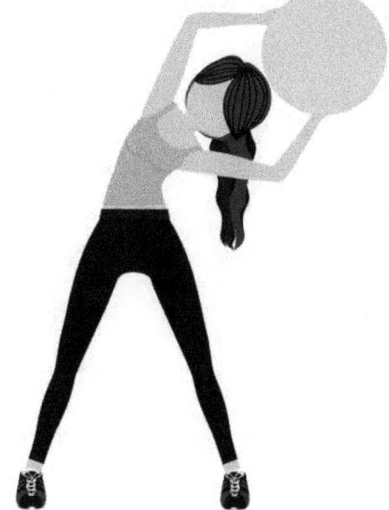

My Food JOURNAL

BREAKFAST:

LUNCH:

DINNER:

CALORIE GOAL **DATE**

My Food DIARY

MEAL	DESCRIPTION	CALORIES	CARBS

Monthly Fitness LOG

FITNESS DIARY

TOP FITNESS GOALS

ACHIEVE

NOTES

Don't forget to hydrate!

MEAL PLAN

BREAKFAST	LUNCH	DINNER

Weekly OVERVIEW

● ● ● ● ● ● ● ● ● ● ● ● ● ● ● ● ●

MONDAY

TUESDAY

WEDNESDAY

THURSDAY

FRIDAY

SATURDAY

SUNDAY

NOTES

Food & Exercise LOG

	BREAKFAST	LUNCH	DINNER	SNACKS	EXERCISE
M					
T					
W					
T					
F					
S					
S					

Food & Exercise LOG

BREAKFAST   **LUNCH**   **DINNER**   **SNACKS**   **EXERCISE**

M

BREAKFAST   **LUNCH**   **DINNER**   **SNACKS**   **EXERCISE**

T

BREAKFAST   **LUNCH**   **DINNER**   **SNACKS**   **EXERCISE**

W

BREAKFAST   **LUNCH**   **DINNER**   **SNACKS**   **EXERCISE**

T

BREAKFAST   **LUNCH**   **DINNER**   **SNACKS**   **EXERCISE**

F

BREAKFAST   **LUNCH**   **DINNER**   **SNACKS**   **EXERCISE**

S

BREAKFAST   **LUNCH**   **DINNER**   **SNACKS**   **EXERCISE**

S

Food & Exercise LOG

	BREAKFAST	LUNCH	DINNER	SNACKS	EXERCISE
M					
T					
W					
T					
F					
S					
S					

Food & Exercise LOG

M | BREAKFAST | LUNCH | DINNER | SNACKS | EXERCISE

T | BREAKFAST | LUNCH | DINNER | SNACKS | EXERCISE

W | BREAKFAST | LUNCH | DINNER | SNACKS | EXERCISE

T | BREAKFAST | LUNCH | DINNER | SNACKS | EXERCISE

F | BREAKFAST | LUNCH | DINNER | SNACKS | EXERCISE

S | BREAKFAST | LUNCH | DINNER | SNACKS | EXERCISE

S | BREAKFAST | LUNCH | DINNER | SNACKS | EXERCISE

February SNAPSHOT

FITNESS PROGRESS PHOTO

MY TOP ACCOMPLISHMENT THIS MONTH

_____
_____
_____
_____
_____

WHAT I HAVE LEARNED

_____
_____
_____

PAIN IS ONLY TEMPORARY BUT VICTORY IS FOREVER

SET YOUR GOALS HIGH AND DON'T STOP TILL YOU GET THERE

WHAT TO DO NEXT MONTH

_____
_____
_____

March SNAPSHOT

MARCH FITNESS GOALS

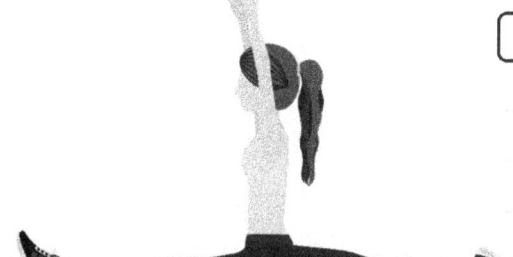

WHAT I WANT TO WORK ON

HOW I WILL REACH MY GOAL

THERE ARE NO Shortcuts TO ANY - PLACE - WORTH GOING

TOP FOCUS OF THE MONTH

NOTES

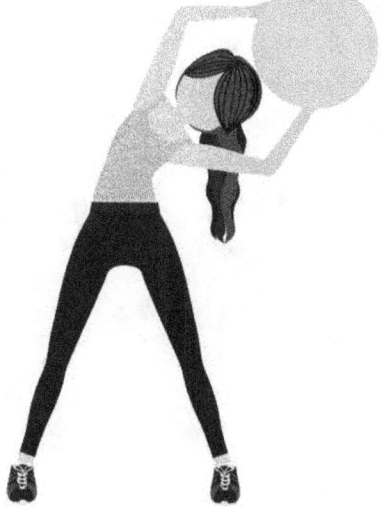

My Food JOURNAL

BREAKFAST:

LUNCH:

DINNER:

CALORIE GOAL **DATE**

My Food DIARY

MEAL	DESCRIPTION	CALORIES	CARBS

Monthly Fitness LOG

FITNESS DIARY

TOP FITNESS GOALS

ACHIEVE

NOTES

Don't forget to hydrate!

MEAL PLAN

BREAKFAST	LUNCH	DINNER

Weekly OVERVIEW

● ● ● ● ● ● ● ● ● ● ● ● ● ● ●

MONDAY

TUESDAY

WEDNESDAY

THURSDAY

FRIDAY

SATURDAY

SUNDAY

NOTES

Food & Exercise LOG

M | BREAKFAST | LUNCH | DINNER | SNACKS | EXERCISE

T | BREAKFAST | LUNCH | DINNER | SNACKS | EXERCISE

W | BREAKFAST | LUNCH | DINNER | SNACKS | EXERCISE

T | BREAKFAST | LUNCH | DINNER | SNACKS | EXERCISE

F | BREAKFAST | LUNCH | DINNER | SNACKS | EXERCISE

S | BREAKFAST | LUNCH | DINNER | SNACKS | EXERCISE

S | BREAKFAST | LUNCH | DINNER | SNACKS | EXERCISE

Food & Exercise LOG

M | BREAKFAST | LUNCH | DINNER | SNACKS | EXERCISE

T | BREAKFAST | LUNCH | DINNER | SNACKS | EXERCISE

W | BREAKFAST | LUNCH | DINNER | SNACKS | EXERCISE

T | BREAKFAST | LUNCH | DINNER | SNACKS | EXERCISE

F | BREAKFAST | LUNCH | DINNER | SNACKS | EXERCISE

S | BREAKFAST | LUNCH | DINNER | SNACKS | EXERCISE

S | BREAKFAST | LUNCH | DINNER | SNACKS | EXERCISE

Food & Exercise LOG

M
BREAKFAST   LUNCH   DINNER   SNACKS   EXERCISE

T
BREAKFAST   LUNCH   DINNER   SNACKS   EXERCISE

W
BREAKFAST   LUNCH   DINNER   SNACKS   EXERCISE

T
BREAKFAST   LUNCH   DINNER   SNACKS   EXERCISE

F
BREAKFAST   LUNCH   DINNER   SNACKS   EXERCISE

S
BREAKFAST   LUNCH   DINNER   SNACKS   EXERCISE

S
BREAKFAST   LUNCH   DINNER   SNACKS   EXERCISE

Food & Exercise LOG

	BREAKFAST	LUNCH	DINNER	SNACKS	EXERCISE
M					
T					
W					
T					
F					
S					
S					

March SNAPSHOT

FITNESS PROGRESS PHOTO

MY TOP ACCOMPLISHMENT THIS MONTH

_____
_____
_____
_____
_____
_____

WHAT I HAVE LEARNED

_____
_____
_____

SET YOUR GOALS **HIGH** AND DON'T STOP **TILL** YOU GET THERE

PAIN IS ONLY **TEMPORARY** BUT VICTORY IS **FOREVER**

WHAT TO DO NEXT MONTH

_____
_____
_____

April SNAPSHOT

APRIL FITNESS GOALS

WHAT I WANT TO WORK ON

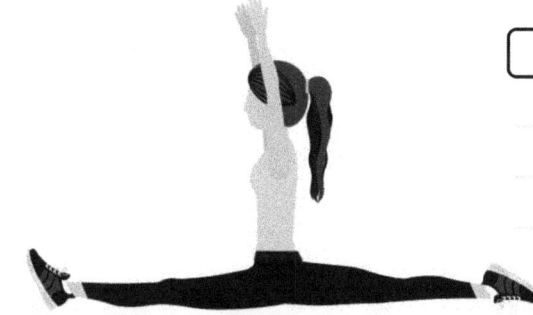

HOW I WILL REACH MY GOAL

THERE ARE NO Shortcuts TO ANY - PLACE - WORTH GOING

TOP FOCUS OF THE MONTH

NOTES

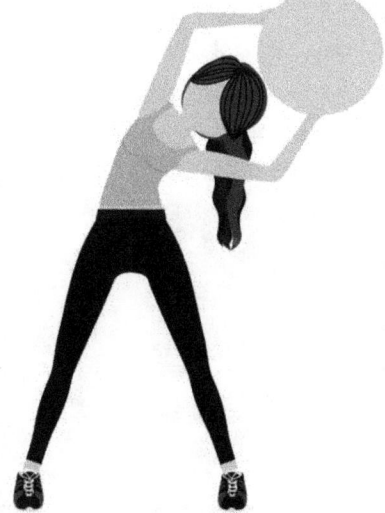

My Food JOURNAL

BREAKFAST:

LUNCH:

DINNER:

CALORIE GOAL   DATE

My Food DIARY

MEAL	DESCRIPTION	CALORIES	CARBS

Monthly Fitness LOG

FITNESS DIARY

TOP FITNESS GOALS

ACHIEVE

NOTES

Don't forget to hydrate!

MEAL PLAN

BREAKFAST	LUNCH	DINNER

Weekly OVERVIEW

● ● ● ● ● ● ● ● ● ● ● ● ● ● ● ●

MONDAY

TUESDAY

WEDNESDAY

THURSDAY

FRIDAY

SATURDAY

SUNDAY

NOTES

Food & Exercise LOG

	BREAKFAST	LUNCH	DINNER	SNACKS	EXERCISE
M					
T					
W					
T					
F					
S					
S					

Food & Exercise LOG

M | BREAKFAST | LUNCH | DINNER | SNACKS | EXERCISE

T | BREAKFAST | LUNCH | DINNER | SNACKS | EXERCISE

W | BREAKFAST | LUNCH | DINNER | SNACKS | EXERCISE

T | BREAKFAST | LUNCH | DINNER | SNACKS | EXERCISE

F | BREAKFAST | LUNCH | DINNER | SNACKS | EXERCISE

S | BREAKFAST | LUNCH | DINNER | SNACKS | EXERCISE

S | BREAKFAST | LUNCH | DINNER | SNACKS | EXERCISE

Food & Exercise LOG

	BREAKFAST	LUNCH	DINNER	SNACKS	EXERCISE
M					
T					
W					
T					
F					
S					
S					

Food & Exercise LOG

M | BREAKFAST | LUNCH | DINNER | SNACKS | EXERCISE

T | BREAKFAST | LUNCH | DINNER | SNACKS | EXERCISE

W | BREAKFAST | LUNCH | DINNER | SNACKS | EXERCISE

T | BREAKFAST | LUNCH | DINNER | SNACKS | EXERCISE

F | BREAKFAST | LUNCH | DINNER | SNACKS | EXERCISE

S | BREAKFAST | LUNCH | DINNER | SNACKS | EXERCISE

S | BREAKFAST | LUNCH | DINNER | SNACKS | EXERCISE

April SNAPSHOT

FITNESS PROGRESS PHOTO

MY TOP ACCOMPLISHMENT THIS MONTH

_____
_____
_____
_____
_____
_____

WHAT I HAVE LEARNED

_____
_____
_____

PAIN IS ONLY TEMPORARY BUT VICTORY IS FOREVER

SET YOUR GOALS HIGH AND DON'T STOP TILL YOU GET THERE

WHAT TO DO NEXT MONTH

_____
_____
_____

May SNAPSHOT

MAY FITNESS GOALS

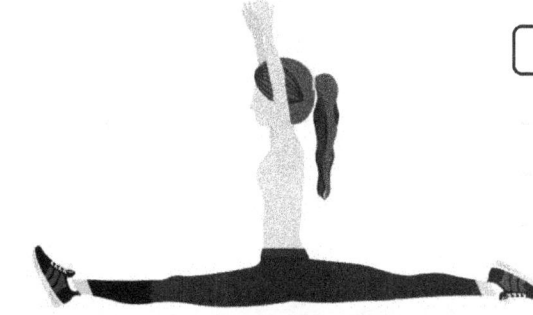

WHAT I WANT TO WORK ON

HOW I WILL REACH MY GOAL

THERE ARE NO *Shortcuts* TO ANY - PLACE - WORTH GOING

TOP FOCUS OF THE MONTH

NOTES

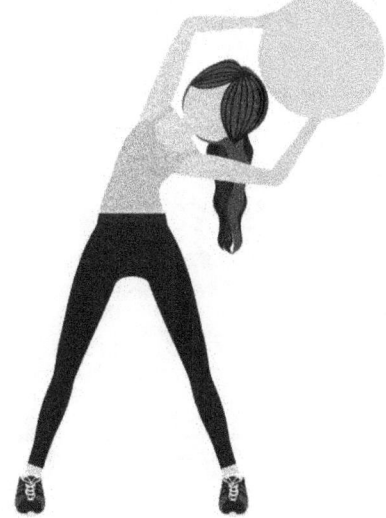

My Food JOURNAL

BREAKFAST:

LUNCH:

DINNER:

CALORIE GOAL		DATE	

My Food DIARY

MEAL	DESCRIPTION	CALORIES	CARBS

Monthly Fitness LOG

FITNESS DIARY

TOP FITNESS GOALS

ACHIEVE

NOTES

Don't forget to hydrate!

MEAL PLAN

BREAKFAST	LUNCH	DINNER

Weekly OVERVIEW

●●●●●●●●●●●●●●●

MONDAY

TUESDAY

WEDNESDAY

THURSDAY

FRIDAY

SATURDAY

SUNDAY

NOTES

Food & Exercise LOG

	BREAKFAST	LUNCH	DINNER	SNACKS	EXERCISE
M					
T					
W					
T					
F					
S					
S					

Food & Exercise LOG

M | BREAKFAST | LUNCH | DINNER | SNACKS | EXERCISE

T | BREAKFAST | LUNCH | DINNER | SNACKS | EXERCISE

W | BREAKFAST | LUNCH | DINNER | SNACKS | EXERCISE

T | BREAKFAST | LUNCH | DINNER | SNACKS | EXERCISE

F | BREAKFAST | LUNCH | DINNER | SNACKS | EXERCISE

S | BREAKFAST | LUNCH | DINNER | SNACKS | EXERCISE

S | BREAKFAST | LUNCH | DINNER | SNACKS | EXERCISE

Food & Exercise LOG

M | BREAKFAST | LUNCH | DINNER | SNACKS | EXERCISE

T | BREAKFAST | LUNCH | DINNER | SNACKS | EXERCISE

W | BREAKFAST | LUNCH | DINNER | SNACKS | EXERCISE

T | BREAKFAST | LUNCH | DINNER | SNACKS | EXERCISE

F | BREAKFAST | LUNCH | DINNER | SNACKS | EXERCISE

S | BREAKFAST | LUNCH | DINNER | SNACKS | EXERCISE

S | BREAKFAST | LUNCH | DINNER | SNACKS | EXERCISE

Food & Exercise LOG

M | BREAKFAST | LUNCH | DINNER | SNACKS | EXERCISE

T | BREAKFAST | LUNCH | DINNER | SNACKS | EXERCISE

W | BREAKFAST | LUNCH | DINNER | SNACKS | EXERCISE

T | BREAKFAST | LUNCH | DINNER | SNACKS | EXERCISE

F | BREAKFAST | LUNCH | DINNER | SNACKS | EXERCISE

S | BREAKFAST | LUNCH | DINNER | SNACKS | EXERCISE

S | BREAKFAST | LUNCH | DINNER | SNACKS | EXERCISE

May SNAPSHOT

FITNESS PROGRESS PHOTO

MY TOP ACCOMPLISHMENT THIS MONTH

_____
_____
_____
_____
_____

WHAT I HAVE LEARNED

_____
_____
_____

PAIN IS ONLY TEMPORARY BUT VICTORY IS FOREVER

SET YOUR GOALS HIGH AND DON'T STOP TILL YOU GET THERE

WHAT TO DO NEXT MONTH

_____
_____
_____

June SNAPSHOT

JUNE FITNESS GOALS

WHAT I WANT TO WORK ON

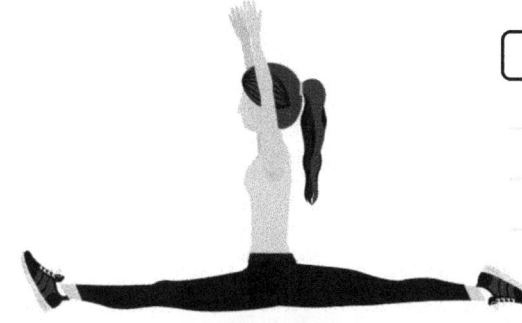

HOW I WILL REACH MY GOAL

THERE ARE NO *Shortcuts* TO ANY - PLACE - WORTH GOING

TOP FOCUS OF THE MONTH

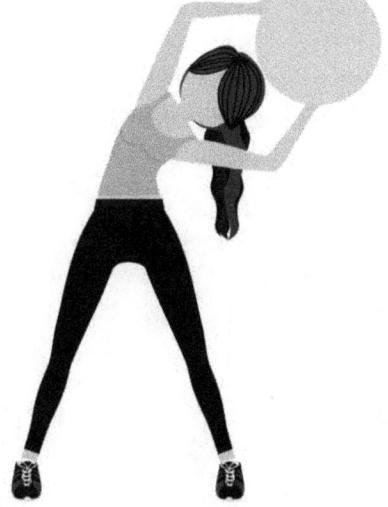

NOTES

My Food JOURNAL

BREAKFAST:

LUNCH:

DINNER:

CALORIE GOAL		DATE	

My Food DIARY

MEAL	DESCRIPTION	CALORIES	CARBS

Monthly Fitness LOG

FITNESS DIARY

TOP FITNESS GOALS

ACHIEVE

NOTES

Don't forget to hydrate!

MEAL PLAN

BREAKFAST	LUNCH	DINNER

Weekly OVERVIEW

●●●●●●●●●●●●●●●

MONDAY

TUESDAY

WEDNESDAY

THURSDAY

FRIDAY

SATURDAY

SUNDAY

NOTES

Food & Exercise LOG

	BREAKFAST	LUNCH	DINNER	SNACKS	EXERCISE
M					
T					
W					
T					
F					
S					
S					

Food & Exercise LOG

M | BREAKFAST | LUNCH | DINNER | SNACKS | EXERCISE

T | BREAKFAST | LUNCH | DINNER | SNACKS | EXERCISE

W | BREAKFAST | LUNCH | DINNER | SNACKS | EXERCISE

T | BREAKFAST | LUNCH | DINNER | SNACKS | EXERCISE

F | BREAKFAST | LUNCH | DINNER | SNACKS | EXERCISE

S | BREAKFAST | LUNCH | DINNER | SNACKS | EXERCISE

S | BREAKFAST | LUNCH | DINNER | SNACKS | EXERCISE

Food & Exercise LOG

M — BREAKFAST · LUNCH · DINNER · SNACKS · EXERCISE

T — BREAKFAST · LUNCH · DINNER · SNACKS · EXERCISE

W — BREAKFAST · LUNCH · DINNER · SNACKS · EXERCISE

T — BREAKFAST · LUNCH · DINNER · SNACKS · EXERCISE

F — BREAKFAST · LUNCH · DINNER · SNACKS · EXERCISE

S — BREAKFAST · LUNCH · DINNER · SNACKS · EXERCISE

S — BREAKFAST · LUNCH · DINNER · SNACKS · EXERCISE

Food & Exercise LOG

	BREAKFAST	LUNCH	DINNER	SNACKS	EXERCISE
M					
T					
W					
T					
F					
S					
S					

June SNAPSHOT

FITNESS PROGRESS PHOTO

MY TOP ACCOMPLISHMENT THIS MONTH

_____
_____
_____
_____
_____

WHAT I HAVE LEARNED

_____
_____
_____

SET YOUR GOALS **HIGH** AND DON'T STOP **TILL** YOU GET THERE

PAIN IS ONLY **TEMPORARY** BUT VICTORY IS **FOREVER**

WHAT TO DO NEXT MONTH

_____
_____
_____

July SNAPSHOT

JULY FITNESS GOALS

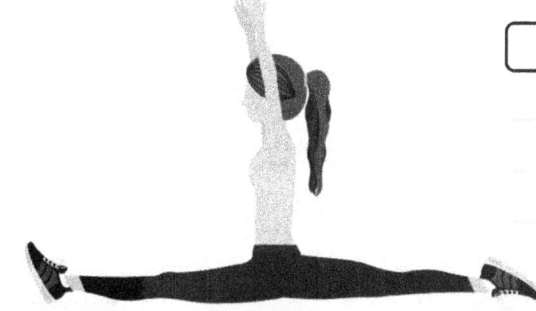

WHAT I WANT TO WORK ON

HOW I WILL REACH MY GOAL

THERE ARE NO Shortcuts TO ANY - PLACE - WORTH GOING

TOP FOCUS OF THE MONTH

NOTES

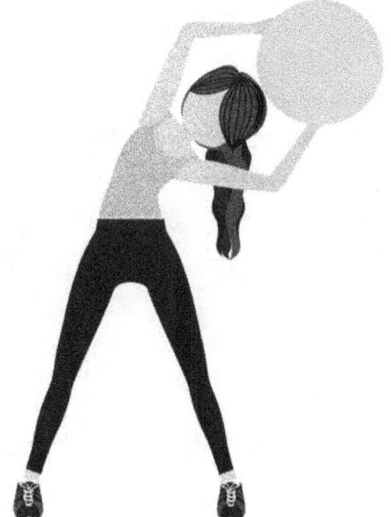

My Food JOURNAL

●●●●●●●●●●●●●

BREAKFAST:

LUNCH:

DINNER:

CALORIE GOAL   DATE

My Food DIARY

MEAL	DESCRIPTION	CALORIES	CARBS

Monthly Fitness LOG

FITNESS DIARY

TOP FITNESS GOALS

ACHIEVE

NOTES

Don't forget to hydrate!

MEAL PLAN

BREAKFAST	LUNCH	DINNER

Weekly OVERVIEW

● ● ● ● ● ● ● ● ● ● ● ● ● ●

MONDAY

TUESDAY

WEDNESDAY

THURSDAY

FRIDAY

SATURDAY

SUNDAY

NOTES

Food & Exercise LOG

M | BREAKFAST | LUNCH | DINNER | SNACKS | EXERCISE

T | BREAKFAST | LUNCH | DINNER | SNACKS | EXERCISE

W | BREAKFAST | LUNCH | DINNER | SNACKS | EXERCISE

T | BREAKFAST | LUNCH | DINNER | SNACKS | EXERCISE

F | BREAKFAST | LUNCH | DINNER | SNACKS | EXERCISE

S | BREAKFAST | LUNCH | DINNER | SNACKS | EXERCISE

S | BREAKFAST | LUNCH | DINNER | SNACKS | EXERCISE

Food & Exercise LOG

	BREAKFAST	LUNCH	DINNER	SNACKS	EXERCISE
M					
T					
W					
T					
F					
S					
S					

Food & Exercise LOG

M — BREAKFAST | LUNCH | DINNER | SNACKS | EXERCISE

T — BREAKFAST | LUNCH | DINNER | SNACKS | EXERCISE

W — BREAKFAST | LUNCH | DINNER | SNACKS | EXERCISE

T — BREAKFAST | LUNCH | DINNER | SNACKS | EXERCISE

F — BREAKFAST | LUNCH | DINNER | SNACKS | EXERCISE

S — BREAKFAST | LUNCH | DINNER | SNACKS | EXERCISE

S — BREAKFAST | LUNCH | DINNER | SNACKS | EXERCISE

Food & Exercise LOG

M | BREAKFAST | LUNCH | DINNER | SNACKS | EXERCISE

T | BREAKFAST | LUNCH | DINNER | SNACKS | EXERCISE

W | BREAKFAST | LUNCH | DINNER | SNACKS | EXERCISE

T | BREAKFAST | LUNCH | DINNER | SNACKS | EXERCISE

F | BREAKFAST | LUNCH | DINNER | SNACKS | EXERCISE

S | BREAKFAST | LUNCH | DINNER | SNACKS | EXERCISE

S | BREAKFAST | LUNCH | DINNER | SNACKS | EXERCISE

July SNAPSHOT

FITNESS PROGRESS PHOTO

MY TOP ACCOMPLISHMENT THIS MONTH

_____
_____
_____
_____
_____

WHAT I HAVE LEARNED

_____
_____

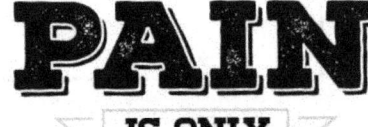

SET YOUR GOALS HIGH AND DON'T STOP TILL YOU GET THERE

PAIN IS ONLY TEMPORARY BUT VICTORY IS FOREVER

WHAT TO DO NEXT MONTH

_____
_____
_____

August SNAPSHOT

AUGUST FITNESS GOALS

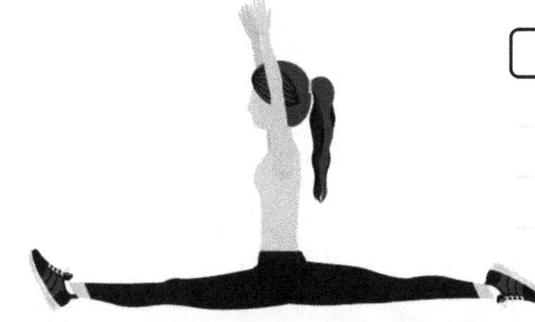

WHAT I WANT TO WORK ON

HOW I WILL REACH MY GOAL

There are no Shortcuts to any place worth going

TOP FOCUS OF THE MONTH

NOTES

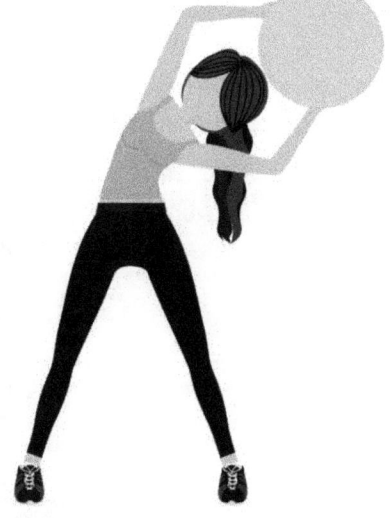

My Food JOURNAL

BREAKFAST:

LUNCH:

DINNER:

CALORIE GOAL | DATE

My Food DIARY

MEAL	DESCRIPTION	CALORIES	CARBS

Monthly Fitness LOG

FITNESS DIARY

TOP FITNESS GOALS

ACHIEVE

NOTES

Don't forget to hydrate!

MEAL PLAN

BREAKFAST	LUNCH	DINNER

Weekly OVERVIEW

● ● ● ● ● ● ● ● ● ● ● ● ● ● ●

MONDAY

TUESDAY

WEDNESDAY

THURSDAY

FRIDAY

SATURDAY

SUNDAY

NOTES

Food & Exercise LOG

M | BREAKFAST | LUNCH | DINNER | SNACKS | EXERCISE

T | BREAKFAST | LUNCH | DINNER | SNACKS | EXERCISE

W | BREAKFAST | LUNCH | DINNER | SNACKS | EXERCISE

T | BREAKFAST | LUNCH | DINNER | SNACKS | EXERCISE

F | BREAKFAST | LUNCH | DINNER | SNACKS | EXERCISE

S | BREAKFAST | LUNCH | DINNER | SNACKS | EXERCISE

S | BREAKFAST | LUNCH | DINNER | SNACKS | EXERCISE

Food & Exercise LOG

	BREAKFAST	LUNCH	DINNER	SNACKS	EXERCISE
M					
T					
W					
T					
F					
S					
S					

Food & Exercise LOG

M | BREAKFAST | LUNCH | DINNER | SNACKS | EXERCISE

T | BREAKFAST | LUNCH | DINNER | SNACKS | EXERCISE

W | BREAKFAST | LUNCH | DINNER | SNACKS | EXERCISE

T | BREAKFAST | LUNCH | DINNER | SNACKS | EXERCISE

F | BREAKFAST | LUNCH | DINNER | SNACKS | EXERCISE

S | BREAKFAST | LUNCH | DINNER | SNACKS | EXERCISE

S | BREAKFAST | LUNCH | DINNER | SNACKS | EXERCISE

Food & Exercise LOG

	BREAKFAST	LUNCH	DINNER	SNACKS	EXERCISE
M					
T					
W					
T					
F					
S					
S					

August SNAPSHOT

FITNESS PROGRESS PHOTO

MY TOP ACCOMPLISHMENT THIS MONTH

_____
_____
_____
_____
_____

WHAT I HAVE LEARNED

_____
_____
_____

PAIN IS ONLY TEMPORARY BUT VICTORY IS FOREVER

SET YOUR GOALS HIGH AND DON'T STOP TILL YOU GET THERE

WHAT TO DO NEXT MONTH

_____
_____
_____

September SNAPSHOT

SEPTEMBER FITNESS GOALS

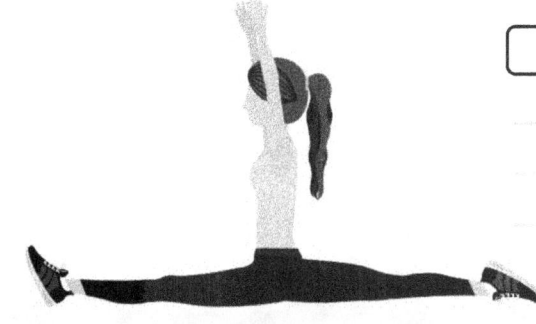

WHAT I WANT TO WORK ON

HOW I WILL REACH MY GOAL

THERE ARE NO Shortcuts TO ANY - PLACE - WORTH GOING

TOP FOCUS OF THE MONTH

NOTES

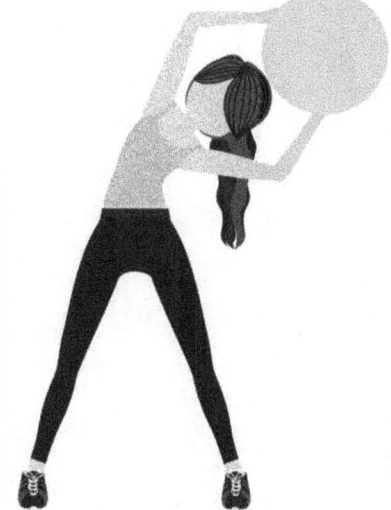

My Food JOURNAL

BREAKFAST:

LUNCH:

DINNER:

CALORIE GOAL **DATE**

My Food DIARY

MEAL	DESCRIPTION	CALORIES	CARBS

Monthly Fitness LOG

FITNESS DIARY

TOP FITNESS GOALS

Achieve

NOTES

Don't forget to hydrate!

MEAL PLAN

BREAKFAST	LUNCH	DINNER

Weekly OVERVIEW

● ● ● ● ● ● ● ● ● ● ● ● ● ● ●

MONDAY

TUESDAY

WEDNESDAY

THURSDAY

FRIDAY

SATURDAY

SUNDAY

NOTES

Food & Exercise LOG

M
BREAKFAST	LUNCH	DINNER	SNACKS	EXERCISE

T
BREAKFAST	LUNCH	DINNER	SNACKS	EXERCISE

W
BREAKFAST	LUNCH	DINNER	SNACKS	EXERCISE

T
BREAKFAST	LUNCH	DINNER	SNACKS	EXERCISE

F
BREAKFAST	LUNCH	DINNER	SNACKS	EXERCISE

S
BREAKFAST	LUNCH	DINNER	SNACKS	EXERCISE

S
BREAKFAST	LUNCH	DINNER	SNACKS	EXERCISE

Food & Exercise LOG

M | BREAKFAST | LUNCH | DINNER | SNACKS | EXERCISE

T | BREAKFAST | LUNCH | DINNER | SNACKS | EXERCISE

W | BREAKFAST | LUNCH | DINNER | SNACKS | EXERCISE

T | BREAKFAST | LUNCH | DINNER | SNACKS | EXERCISE

F | BREAKFAST | LUNCH | DINNER | SNACKS | EXERCISE

S | BREAKFAST | LUNCH | DINNER | SNACKS | EXERCISE

S | BREAKFAST | LUNCH | DINNER | SNACKS | EXERCISE

Food & Exercise LOG

	BREAKFAST	LUNCH	DINNER	SNACKS	EXERCISE
M					
T					
W					
T					
F					
S					
S					

Food & Exercise LOG

M — BREAKFAST | LUNCH | DINNER | SNACKS | EXERCISE

T — BREAKFAST | LUNCH | DINNER | SNACKS | EXERCISE

W — BREAKFAST | LUNCH | DINNER | SNACKS | EXERCISE

T — BREAKFAST | LUNCH | DINNER | SNACKS | EXERCISE

F — BREAKFAST | LUNCH | DINNER | SNACKS | EXERCISE

S — BREAKFAST | LUNCH | DINNER | SNACKS | EXERCISE

S — BREAKFAST | LUNCH | DINNER | SNACKS | EXERCISE

September SNAPSHOT

FITNESS PROGRESS PHOTO

MY TOP ACCOMPLISHMENT THIS MONTH

_____
_____
_____
_____
_____
_____

WHAT I HAVE LEARNED

_____
_____

PAIN IS ONLY TEMPORARY BUT VICTORY IS FOREVER

SET YOUR GOALS HIGH AND DON'T STOP TILL YOU GET THERE

WHAT TO DO NEXT MONTH

_____
_____

October SNAPSHOT

OCTOBER FITNESS GOALS

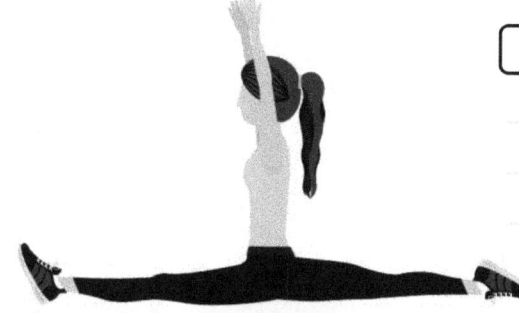

WHAT I WANT TO WORK ON

HOW I WILL REACH MY GOAL

THERE ARE NO Shortcuts TO ANY - PLACE - WORTH GOING

TOP FOCUS OF THE MONTH

NOTES

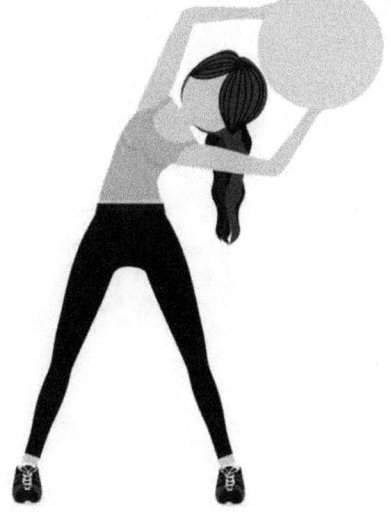

My Food JOURNAL

BREAKFAST:

LUNCH:

DINNER:

CALORIE GOAL   DATE

My Food DIARY

MEAL	DESCRIPTION	CALORIES	CARBS

Monthly Fitness LOG

FITNESS DIARY

TOP FITNESS GOALS

ACHIEVE

NOTES

Don't forget to hydrate!

MEAL PLAN

BREAKFAST	LUNCH	DINNER

Weekly OVERVIEW

● ● ● ● ● ● ● ● ● ● ● ● ● ● ● ● ●

MONDAY

TUESDAY

WEDNESDAY

THURSDAY

FRIDAY

SATURDAY

SUNDAY

NOTES

Food & Exercise LOG

	BREAKFAST	LUNCH	DINNER	SNACKS	EXERCISE
M					
T					
W					
T					
F					
S					
S					

Food & Exercise LOG

	BREAKFAST	LUNCH	DINNER	SNACKS	EXERCISE
M					
T					
W					
T					
F					
S					
S					

Food & Exercise LOG

M
BREAKFAST | LUNCH | DINNER | SNACKS | EXERCISE

T
BREAKFAST | LUNCH | DINNER | SNACKS | EXERCISE

W
BREAKFAST | LUNCH | DINNER | SNACKS | EXERCISE

T
BREAKFAST | LUNCH | DINNER | SNACKS | EXERCISE

F
BREAKFAST | LUNCH | DINNER | SNACKS | EXERCISE

S
BREAKFAST | LUNCH | DINNER | SNACKS | EXERCISE

S
BREAKFAST | LUNCH | DINNER | SNACKS | EXERCISE

Food & Exercise LOG

M | BREAKFAST | LUNCH | DINNER | SNACKS | EXERCISE

T | BREAKFAST | LUNCH | DINNER | SNACKS | EXERCISE

W | BREAKFAST | LUNCH | DINNER | SNACKS | EXERCISE

T | BREAKFAST | LUNCH | DINNER | SNACKS | EXERCISE

F | BREAKFAST | LUNCH | DINNER | SNACKS | EXERCISE

S | BREAKFAST | LUNCH | DINNER | SNACKS | EXERCISE

S | BREAKFAST | LUNCH | DINNER | SNACKS | EXERCISE

October SNAPSHOT

FITNESS PROGRESS PHOTO

MY TOP ACCOMPLISHMENT THIS MONTH

_____
_____
_____
_____
_____
_____

WHAT I HAVE LEARNED

_____
_____
_____

PAIN IS ONLY TEMPORARY BUT VICTORY IS FOREVER

SET YOUR GOALS HIGH AND DON'T STOP TILL YOU GET THERE

WHAT TO DO NEXT MONTH

_____
_____
_____

November SNAPSHOT

NOVEMBER FITNESS GOALS

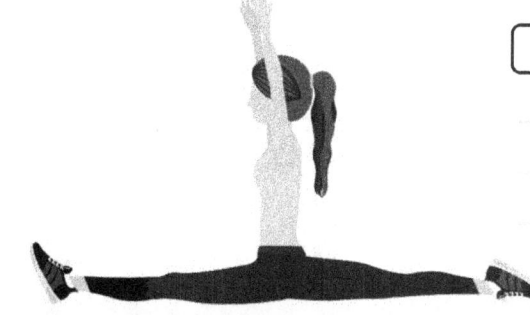

WHAT I WANT TO WORK ON

HOW I WILL REACH MY GOAL

THERE ARE NO Shortcuts TO ANY - PLACE - WORTH GOING

TOP FOCUS OF THE MONTH

NOTES

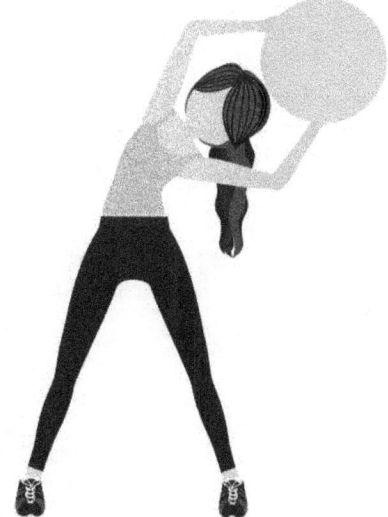

My Food JOURNAL

BREAKFAST:

LUNCH:

DINNER:

CALORIE GOAL **DATE**

My Food DIARY

MEAL	DESCRIPTION	CALORIES	CARBS

Monthly Fitness LOG

FITNESS DIARY

TOP FITNESS GOALS

Achieve

NOTES

Don't forget to hydrate!

MEAL PLAN

BREAKFAST	LUNCH	DINNER

Weekly OVERVIEW

● ● ● ● ● ● ● ● ● ● ● ● ● ● ●

MONDAY

TUESDAY

WEDNESDAY

THURSDAY

FRIDAY

SATURDAY

SUNDAY

NOTES

Food & Exercise LOG

	BREAKFAST	LUNCH	DINNER	SNACKS	EXERCISE
M					
T					
W					
T					
F					
S					
S					

Food & Exercise LOG

M | BREAKFAST | LUNCH | DINNER | SNACKS | EXERCISE

T | BREAKFAST | LUNCH | DINNER | SNACKS | EXERCISE

W | BREAKFAST | LUNCH | DINNER | SNACKS | EXERCISE

T | BREAKFAST | LUNCH | DINNER | SNACKS | EXERCISE

F | BREAKFAST | LUNCH | DINNER | SNACKS | EXERCISE

S | BREAKFAST | LUNCH | DINNER | SNACKS | EXERCISE

S | BREAKFAST | LUNCH | DINNER | SNACKS | EXERCISE

Food & Exercise LOG

	BREAKFAST	LUNCH	DINNER	SNACKS	EXERCISE
M					
T					
W					
T					
F					
S					
S					

Food & Exercise LOG

M | BREAKFAST | LUNCH | DINNER | SNACKS | EXERCISE

T | BREAKFAST | LUNCH | DINNER | SNACKS | EXERCISE

W | BREAKFAST | LUNCH | DINNER | SNACKS | EXERCISE

T | BREAKFAST | LUNCH | DINNER | SNACKS | EXERCISE

F | BREAKFAST | LUNCH | DINNER | SNACKS | EXERCISE

S | BREAKFAST | LUNCH | DINNER | SNACKS | EXERCISE

S | BREAKFAST | LUNCH | DINNER | SNACKS | EXERCISE

November SNAPSHOT

FITNESS PROGRESS PHOTO

MY TOP ACCOMPLISHMENT THIS MONTH

_____
_____
_____
_____
_____

WHAT I HAVE LEARNED

_____
_____
_____

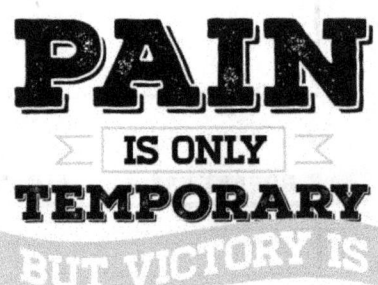

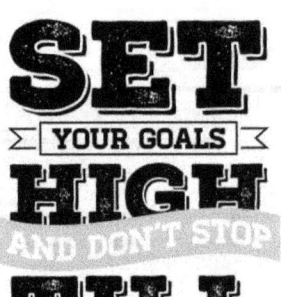

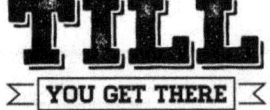

WHAT TO DO NEXT MONTH

_____
_____
_____

December SNAPSHOT

DECEMBER FITNESS GOALS

WHAT I WANT TO WORK ON

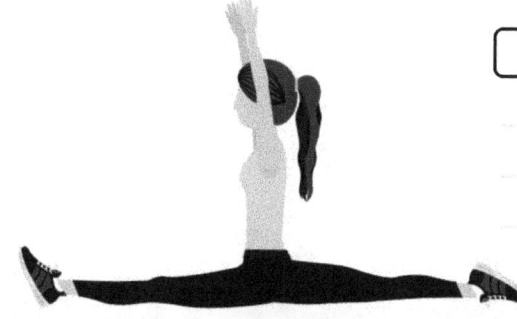

HOW I WILL REACH MY GOAL

THERE ARE NO Shortcuts TO ANY - PLACE - WORTH GOING

TOP FOCUS OF THE MONTH

NOTES

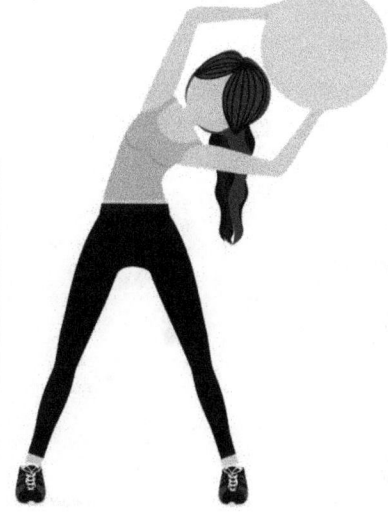

My Food JOURNAL

BREAKFAST:

LUNCH:

DINNER:

CALORIE GOAL | DATE

My Food DIARY

MEAL	DESCRIPTION	CALORIES	CARBS

Monthly Fitness LOG

●●●●●●●●●●●

FITNESS DIARY

TOP FITNESS GOALS

ACHIEVE

NOTES

Don't forget to hydrate! ○○○○ ○○○○

MEAL PLAN

BREAKFAST	LUNCH	DINNER

Weekly OVERVIEW

MONDAY

TUESDAY

WEDNESDAY

THURSDAY

FRIDAY

SATURDAY

SUNDAY

NOTES

Food & Exercise LOG

	BREAKFAST	LUNCH	DINNER	SNACKS	EXERCISE
M					
T					
W					
T					
F					
S					
S					

Food & Exercise LOG

	BREAKFAST	LUNCH	DINNER	SNACKS	EXERCISE
M					
T					
W					
T					
F					
S					
S					

Food & Exercise LOG

M | BREAKFAST | LUNCH | DINNER | SNACKS | EXERCISE

T | BREAKFAST | LUNCH | DINNER | SNACKS | EXERCISE

W | BREAKFAST | LUNCH | DINNER | SNACKS | EXERCISE

T | BREAKFAST | LUNCH | DINNER | SNACKS | EXERCISE

F | BREAKFAST | LUNCH | DINNER | SNACKS | EXERCISE

S | BREAKFAST | LUNCH | DINNER | SNACKS | EXERCISE

S | BREAKFAST | LUNCH | DINNER | SNACKS | EXERCISE

Food & Exercise LOG

	BREAKFAST	LUNCH	DINNER	SNACKS	EXERCISE
M					
T					
W					
T					
F					
S					
S					

December SNAPSHOT

FITNESS PROGRESS PHOTO

MY TOP ACCOMPLISHMENT THIS MONTH

_____
_____
_____
_____
_____

WHAT I HAVE LEARNED

_____
_____
_____

SET YOUR GOALS HIGH AND DON'T STOP TILL YOU GET THERE

PAIN IS ONLY TEMPORARY BUT VICTORY IS FOREVER

WHAT TO DO NEXT MONTH

_____
_____
_____

Workout IDEAS

| JAN | FEB | MAR | APR | MAY | JUN | JUL | AUG | SEP | OCT | NOV | DEC |

EXERCISE / WORK OUT IDEAS

NOTES

Workout IDEAS

JAN　FEB　MAR　APR　MAY　JUN　JUL　AUG　SEP　OCT　NOV　DEC

EXERCISE / WORK OUT IDEAS	NOTES

Workout IDEAS

| JAN | FEB | MAR | APR | MAY | JUN | JUL | AUG | SEP | OCT | NOV | DEC |

EXERCISE / WORK OUT IDEAS | **NOTES**

Workout IDEAS

| JAN | FEB | MAR | APR | MAY | JUN | JUL | AUG | SEP | OCT | NOV | DEC |

EXERCISE / WORK OUT IDEAS | **NOTES**

Fitness DIARY

Fitness DIARY

Fitness DIARY

Fitness DIARY

Fitness DIARY

Fitness DIARY

Fitness DIARY

Fitness DIARY

Fitness DIARY

Fitness DIARY

Fitness DIARY

Fitness DIARY

Fitness DIARY

Fitness DIARY

www.ingramcontent.com/pod-product-compliance
Lightning Source LLC
Chambersburg PA
CBHW080214040426
42333CB00044B/2675